Macrobiotic Diet Cookbook

50+ Macrobiotic Recipes for Holistic Wellness and High Energy Levels

Written by Marta Tuchowska

Copyright Marta Tuchowska & Holistic Wellness Project Ltd. © 2014, 2016

www.holisticwellnessproject.com

All cooking is an experiment in a sense, and many people come to the same or similar recipe over time. All recipes in this book have been derived from author's personal experience. Should any bear a close resemblance to those used elsewhere, that is purely coincidental.

The book is not intended to provide medical advice or to take the place of medical advice and treatment from your personal physician. Readers are advised to consult their own doctors or other qualified health professionals regarding the treatment of medical conditions. The author shall not be held liable or responsible for any misunderstanding or misuse of the information contained in this book. The information is not intended to diagnose, treat or cure any disease.

It is important to remember that the author of this book is not a doctor/ medical professional. Only opinions based upon her own personal experiences or research are cited. THE AUTHOR DOES NOT OFFER MEDICAL ADVICE or prescribe any treatments. For any health or medical issues – you should be talking to your doctor first.

Contents

A Few Words about Me and This Book

Thank you for purchasing my book. It really means a lot to me. My goal is to familiarize you, the reader, with the various benefits of a macrobiotic diet in a 100% practical way. This is why the macrobiotic style recipes are the main focus of this book. I am sure that they can help you feel more energized and happier in your body. The way I always put it myself: *you will be experiencing wellness in a holistic way.*

If this is your first time reading one of my books, let me briefly introduce myself. My name is Marta, I am 32 years old (as of 2015) and to cut a long story short- I am a real wellness freak.

I have always felt attracted to a healthy lifestyle, natural therapies, yoga, and fitness. It's just a part of who I am, I guess. I can't live in a different way. On my way to achieving wellness, I have also encountered various obstacles, like for example falling off track, unhealthy temptations usually provoked by lack of motivation.

I struggled with no zest and no energy for life and felt a bit trapped in diets that did not work and made me feel sick, tired and disappointed. It wasn't until I said "enough of that" and decided to focus on long-term solutions and took care of my mind and body in a truly holistic way.

This is what I want to show you in this book. It's all interconnected: the way you eat, feel, think, make decisions, and take care of yourself.

As a part of my wellness journey, I studied naturopathy, aromatherapy, and other natural therapies, as well as, of course, holistic nutrition.

Finally, I managed to change my career and move it into direction I wanted to, which of course, was wellness and helping others achieve it.

Even though, originally I trained in massage therapy and studied the human body, and imagined that it would be my ultimate goal, it turned out to be simply a drop in the ocean of wellness and health creativity I was just about to dive into. Lesson number one that I learned while offering massage treatments was that people wanted to learn more about self-care, nutrition, balancing their energy levels, and that it really wasn't only about massage. Most of my clients would ask me about a type of a diet I was following, what to eat, how to relax at home to prevent pain and finally (and most importantly!)- HOW TO HAVE MORE ENERGY on a daily basis.

21st century people always complain about low energy levels, and even if they don't, they wish they had more energy to get more stuff done.

Nutrition is the basics of the health foundation you can create for yourself. Then, there is also motivation. This is why I am also currently involved in coaching. Not only wellness coaching, but also motivational and lifestyle coaching.

I have always enjoyed motivating people and helping them live their lives to the fullest. Making them realize that they can achieve their goals and be the creators of their lives. Health is the number one lesson you will have to learn. Remember, no one else is going to do it for you.

You have a certain responsibility here. It's going be fun though. Healthy eating means a strong body and a focused mind. It also means that you will be inspiring those around you. What more can you ask for?

This is my objective. Every day, I aim to create more amazingly healthy habits for myself so that I can inspire other people.

I want to help you take action in a practical way.

As Stephan R.Covey, the author of the book "The Seven Habits of Highly Effective People", says "To know and not to do is really not to know".

This is why I have created HolisticWellnessProject.com where I share a myriad of simple, practical, yet effective wellness and personal development tips that hopefully can help you create your own holistic lifestyle you love.

How I got started on the Macrobiotic Diet

My favorite nutritional patterns that work well for me are pretty much plant-based, vegan/vegetarian I am a firm believer in the Alkaline Diet (I also love raw vegan foods) and it is really similar to the Macrobiotic Diet. In fact, if you follow the Macrobiotic Diet, you could also say that you eat pretty much alkaline.

I also believe that even if you don't want to go fully plant-based at this stage of your life, you can still benefit a lot simply from reducing animal products. It's as simple as that.

BEFORE WE START:
- I am not telling you what to do. No preaching. Never. I am telling you what I do. I am not a guru. I am a do-ro. I am here to share my preferred eating patterns and recipes so that you can create your own way. Everyone

is different- this is the foundation of every holistic therapy or approach there is.

- This is not a weight loss program or any dietary program. I am not a fan of the same programs with the same "proven steps and strategies" for everyone. If you stick with the Macrobiotic way, you will give your body more nutrients, and eliminate empty calories and foods with no real nutritional values. You will also detoxify your body in a natural way. That's the best, natural "weight loss program" that you can treat your body with.

- One thing is sure, if you are interested in or following the alkaline diet, the plant-based diet, the vegetarian diet, then the Macrobiotic Kingdom of healthy cooking is something for you to explore. Macrobiotic way is definitely a party that you want to be at.

- If you are Paleo, then this may not be the book for you. We are using grains and legumes here at our Macrobiotic party. But...you are more than welcome to join our boat....Just try it and see what works for you. It's always good to relax and enjoy something new!

From my own experience, when it comes to grains and legumes, I think that one needs to test which ones suit them. For example, I love quinoa, millet, and amaranth. They agree with my stomach, but I also listen to my body. However, I know people who are allergic to certain types of grains (even though the grains are integral, organic, and only minimally processed).

The same with legumes, I know many vegans who eat legumes on a daily basis and don't develop any digestive problems. However, my stomach does not tolerate large amounts of legumes. I can use them in salads, or mixed with some healthy grains like quinoa and I am fine. It's good to try different ways, listen to your body, and observe its reactions. Don't jump on any band wagons, create your own and be the driver- I am like a broken record with that. Variety and balance is the key to success.

The Macrobiotic Way

After having tried numerous types of diets myself, it gives me great pleasure to introduce this amazing diet that can help in restoring your energy levels and finding a new, balanced version of yourself.

I first heard about the Macrobiotic Diet back in 2009 when I lived in Italy. My friend's wife mentioned this diet to me as she thought I would get interested in it. And I did! I really did. I did some research online but found lots of information that was just too much for me to take in. Yin and yang- it was something I was not familiar with and so, I mistakenly thought that it was too complicated and that there was no place for me to join the Macrobiotic cooking party at that point.

But it did attract my attention. Roberta, my friend's wife, was about 45 years old (and a mother of 4) but she looked like 27-28. Yes! She said she had been following the macrobiotic diet ever since she was 30. Apparently, it helped her lose weight after having her first baby.

After moving back to Spain, I decided to join a few Macrobiotic Diet workshops and learn more. Again, I found the classes too theoretical and so I did not take action really. I really think that when it comes to exploring new diets, the best you can do first is to get as many recipes as you can and try them. Then you can dive more into theory.

Finally, I got a few books written by a famous Spanish naturopath, Dr. Jorge Pérez-Calvo Soler. It was more theory again but there were also a few practical guidelines and recipes and so I could finally get my feet wet in Macrobiotic, energizing cuisine. It also coincided with my research in the Alkaline Diet, something that is not really that well-known here Spain. What's really trendy here now (as of 2015) is the Macrobiotic Diet.

I also attended a few macrobiotic cooking workshops and, being as practical a person as I am, I finally felt like fish in the water! I felt progress. I cooked, I ate, I tried new recipes, I observed my body, and started to make my own conclusions. This is why I have written this book. It's based on my personal experiences with my Macrobiotic cooking "experiments" from the past 3 years.

There is also a big Alkaline influence, since it is the main approach that I follow. Like I said before, these two diets very often overlap and they both promote eliminating or reducing animal products as well as adding more fresh vegetables into your diet. *Hmm...looks like we have heard it before.* But...have we actually taken action? If not, it was probably as we did not know what to eat and how to create recipes that keeps us inspired and satisfied. But no worries...with this book, we got you fully covered!

If you are new to the Alkaline Diet, I offer an Alkaline Wellness email newsletter, you can sign up for at no cost by visiting the link below:

www.holisticwellnessproject.com/alkaline

Oh, and when you sign up, you will receive free instant access to these VIP Bonus guides:

3 Free Bonus Guides

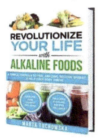 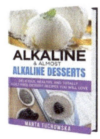 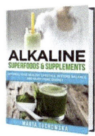

That's plenty of recipes and information to make sure you are making progress and restoring energy and health you deserve! (any problems with your sign-up, be sure to email me at: info@holisticwellnessproject.com)

I like comparing different diets. Of course, the Macrobiotic diet is much more complex than the Alkaline Diet. The Macrobiotic Diet is an oriental therapy, and so in order to adjust it to your own case, or try to heal certain ailments that you may be suffering from, the Macrobiotic Diet practitioner would take into account your geographical location, the season, ethnicity, and which organs need cleansing or nourishing so that the body can heal itself and much, much more.

My recipes offer a general overview of the Macrobiotic cooking for beginners.

I want to show you how much variety, taste, and pleasure you can put into the Macrobiotic Diet without having to investigate its rather complicated (but also extremely interesting) theory to begin with.

I promise that this book will make it much easier for you to cook Macrobiotic meals and see the results for yourself. I also hope that this book will change your perspective about the Macrobiotic Diet and make cooking more enjoyable in general. I very often spend long hours in my kitchen.

I love creating and learning new things. While cooking, I usually listen to music, and motivational podcasts and videos. I enjoy feeding my brain with positive stuff while preparing my food. I think it creates some kind of energy, would you agree with me? Music that puts me in a good mood as well as all kinds of "motivational stuff" - it all creates an incredible atmosphere that I look forward to. This is how I do it. You may also want to do the same or adjust it to your own taste.

One thing I learned- if you want to learn healthy cooking- your kitchen should be your temple. What I also draw pleasure and satisfaction from is cooking for the people I love.

Ok, back to the Macrobiotic Diet as this is why we are here, right?

Macrobiotic Diet - Comprehend the Basics

Let us begin with understanding the concept of the Macrobiotic Diet. Here are a few interesting facts:

- This diet was introduced by a German doctor named Hufeland. He wrote a book in 1797, where he talked about the different the ways to increase the longevity of human life.

- According to Hufeland, the concept of a macrobiotic diet is not just a means to cure diseases; it was a way to increase the life span of human beings. Recently, authors like Simon Browne have stated that the Macrobiotic Diet is an approach that heals the body's health along with the mind and soul.

- The Japanese military doctor Shagen Ishizuka and macrobiotics theorist George Oshawa go as far as bringing in the concept of Yin and Yang (more on that in my future books for sure, like I said this is just a simple cookbook) of the Japanese philosophy to describe the diet. This diet is majorly centered on the concept of balancing the required food items in a healthy manner without exceeding the intake.

- It focuses on consuming substantial amount of green vegetables and grains. The entire concept of the Macrobiotic Diet is built on the concept of eating only when you are hungry. It stresses upon the fact that one should eat in moderation. Just like the yogi philosophy says: after eating your meal, you should feel nicely energized, and your body and mind should feel fueled, not lethargic.

- Food that is hard to digest like meat, animal fat, poultry or dairy products, chocolates, vanilla, strong alcoholic beverages, foods with preservatives and other highly processed foods, should be avoided in the macrobiotic dietary system (just like on the alkaline diet).

- The Macrobiotic Diet recommends that food should be minimally cooked, in order to retain its natural nutrition. So here, we can say that if pretty much overlaps with the raw foods philosophy hence allowing us receive more vital nutrients in our diet.

- The Macrobiotic Diet doesn't just focus on what we eat; after all it is a holistic, oriental therapy. It focuses on the overall lifestyle of a person. It promotes a healthy outlook towards life; like exercising regularly, getting less involved with the television or the computer, spending time outdoors and rebalancing oneself with nature (since I have chosen to live in the countryside, I get to enjoy this natural rebalancing therapy daily, plus it's free, the best spa ever!).

Still, if you lack energy, and most of us- with our 21st century lifestyles- do or did at some point, the least thing you can think of is to move your body, get off the couch, and go to the gym or do yoga. This is why the first step that I always recommend to anyone complaining from low energy levels is to have a closer look at one's nutrition. Of course, don't forget to get a checkup by your doctor, if you're always tired, you may be lacking some vitamins, minerals or be suffering from some disease; remember not to neglect regular checkups, even if you believe in natural/holistic medicine, like I do. Standard medicine should not be rejected.

Lack of time, yes I know! I totally understand. But...

Less activity is better than no activity.

It doesn't have to be ALL OR NOTHING. Find balance that works for you.

It's more about easy and sustainable habits.

So, if you don't have time for super long everyday workouts, just commit to short, 10 minutes workouts. Your efforts will compound! Besides, it's easy to trick your brain by saying- OK, all I need to do is to work out for 5-10 minutes before my morning/evening shower. Sound good?

The same with healthy cooking. I learned to cook in bulk, freeze, and plan my meals so as not to waste any of my time. It's your brain that tries to come up with excuses, and it always will. You need to make a decision to outsmart it.

How can busy, stressed out, 21st century individuals benefit from the Macrobiotic Diet?

The Macrobiotic Diet is becoming increasingly popular in the Western countries. People need balance, it's as simple as that. The SAD diet (Standard American Diet) is also taking its toll outside of the United States (let's call it the Standard Western Diet).

Lack of time, globalization, and a myriad of typical excuses of "but I..." that people normally come up with are to blame. I get it, I have been there myself. The good news is that it's time to focus on solutions that work and can help you create a stronger, happier and more balanced version of yourself. The natural, Macrobiotic approach can help save the world, and make it a happier place.

The Macrobiotic Diet's goal is moderation and a healthy lifestyle. It is highly recommended for our competitive and stressful lives, as it aids in physical, spiritual and mental development.

When you feel good in your body, you also feel happier and more focused. In other words- less annoyed and more balanced.

The Associated Lifestyle

The Macrobiotic lifestyle is not simply about following a diet chart - it is a holistic approach to a better lifestyle. It's about eating in a natural way, optimizing the process of digestion (making it easier for our digestive system). It makes the body stronger, improves the immunity system, and keeps body weight in check.

Here are some of the benefits that you can reap for yourself.

You can reduce weight and keep fit

Health and wellness freaks who have been following stringent fad diets can find a good alternative by adopting a Macrobiotic lifestyle. This is because the Macrobiotic Diet is largely composed of food items that have a low-GI, low fat, and high fiber content.

This diet has a double advantage —it doesn't just contribute towards the nourishment of the body; it also helps achieve mental harmony. Along with consuming seasonal food items, the Macrobiotic Diet excludes all processed foods, thus creating balance and harmony between our body and nature.

You can Ease PMS and other female ailments (I managed!)

The Macrobiotic Diet has an additional benefit for women. This diet, being rich in phytoestrogens, is especially helpful for women who suffer from premenstrual syndrome. It helps women get relief from menopausal symptoms. It is also beneficial to women suffering from endometriosis, which causes painful periods. My mom managed to reduce all the unwanted menopausal symptoms utilizing the balanced, Macrobiotic Diet and so she did not need to rely on hormone pills.

From my own experience: the first thing that I recommend for you to ease PMS (or if you are a guy reading this, then you may pass it on to your wife or girlfriend- you will not suffer while she suffers, if you know what I mean) is to quit coffee and caffeine in general. As simple as it is, it is extremely effective. We were not designed to get our energy from caffeine. Moreover, caffeine deprives us of magnesium and iron.
Use roibosh tea and kukicha tea instead. Add some almond milk. It will energize you in a natural way, you won't need caffeine.

Society and commercial main-stream marketing sell us many things that we apparently need (including coffee) but the truth is that we don't.

The reason why I mention this is that the Macrobiotic Diet also encourages us to be conscious about what we do and about our everyday choices. The way I always put it myself is "Brainstorming-yes! Brainwashing-no!". Try to question everything you see and experience. The fact that everyone does this or that does not mean that a given activity is good for you.

I know that quitting coffee can be a long process, for some people it is as difficult as giving up smoking or even worse. I used to be addicted to coffee and it was really hard for me to quit it. My final tip for you is- see what works for you. Even if you decide to reduce coffee and add more herbal infusions or natural green juices instead, you will enjoy higher energy levels and more zest for life.

Try it. Test it. I don't want to preach to you. I know that coffee is really hard to quit and all I want to do is to help you feel more energetic in a natural way. "Just try to reduce it if you don't want to quit it"- is a great place to start! (works not only for coffee). Again, we don't need to torture ourselves with all or nothing mentality.

Youthful look and healthy skin

Essential vitamins present in fruits and vegetables contribute towards a great complexion. If followed for a long term, the macrobiotic diet can prevent premature ageing, keeping the body fit, and will lower the risk of heart disease.

Prevention and control of diabetes (great branch of complementary medicine)

Several researchers have unanimously observed that being overweight is directly linked to the augmentation of the risk of developing Type 2 diabetes. Since the Macrobiotic Diet is beneficial in keeping body weight in check and preventing obesity, following such a lifestyle is very likely to reduce the chances of becoming diabetic.

Apart from prevention of diabetes, macrobiotic diet is also good for people already suffering from diabetes as it helps in keeping the disease in control. A study conducted on a small sample group showed that when people with type 2 diabetes followed a Macrobiotic Diet, they showed significantly lower levels of A1C.

Of course, if you are diabetic, I suggest you consult all changes in your diet with your doctor.

Healthy cardiovascular system

The levels of triglycerides (a fatty substance in blood) and cholesterol have been associated with the risk of heart disease. The Macrobiotic Diet being devoid of processed food and consisting of grains and fiber constitutes of what has been universally accepted as heart-friendly diet, keeping the cholesterol level and blood pressure in check.

Preparing To Go Macrobiotic- What Do You Need?

Now that you have decided to go Macrobiotic (this is what I am hoping), you must keep in mind the ingredients that form the basis of a Macrobiotic meal and the ingredients that you should try to avoid. The basic principle of a Macrobiotic meal is to have a nutritious and well balanced diet. So here is a list of ingredients that will form your Macrobiotic meal. It's time to equip your kitchen!

Grains

Brown rice is important for a Macrobiotic Diet. Keep both the kinds of short and long grains as short grains are considered to be more nutritious than long grains but are stickier. Quinoa, rolled oats, millet, and barley are also popular grains. You can also use wild rice or even black rice in your Macrobiotic Diet along with wehani. Yam, Buckwheat, or lotus root soba noodles can be used as a base for a quick meal. Udon noodles are used in soups. You can also choose gluten-free versions, or naturally gluten-free grains such as quinoa (my favorite).

Beans and Pulses

Beans and pulses also form the basis of a Macrobiotic Diet. Adzuki (aduki), black, northern, kidney, pinto, mung, chickpeas, and split peas, red, green and black lentils - all have a lot of nutritional value. Kombu seaweed or bay leaf, when added during cooking will aid digestion.

Sea Vegetables

Sea vegetables are proved to be a rich source of minerals. They are speculated to have the power to heal and restore balance. A nutritious alternative to gelatin could be agar-agar. Arame, kombuhijiki, dulse, nori, and wakame can be used in sauces, stir-fry, salads, and soups. Hijiki should be avoided by expectant or nursing women as it is high in mercury.

Seasonings

Sea salt, shoyu, miso, or soy sauce are amazing macrobiotic seasonings. Rice vinegar (brown) and sesame oil should also be invited to your kitchen. Gomasio, umeboshi plum vinegar, natural sauerkraut and dried shiitake will add a new dimension to your cooking.

Sweeteners

Macrobiotic sweeteners include rice syrup, maple syrup, and barley malt. Agave nectar can be used as a viable alternative. It is completely unrefined, low glycemic, and an excellent sweetener.

What I use (if I really need to): stevia, and...bananas. Yes, they are super sweet!

Beverages

Bancha tea is type of green tea that is very healthy and apt for this diet. Kukicha, or twig tea, is a blend of green tea that has a mildly nutty flavor, has a low caffeine quota and high antioxidant quota. A substitute for coffee is Roasted Barley, which is slightly bitter in taste. Teecino is also used in a Macrobiotic Diet. It has a rich flavor palette. Peppermint and Ginger teas facilitate digestion. I suggest you experiment with as many herbal, caffeine-free infusions as you can. They will restore your energy naturally.

Clean water (use filters, avoid tap water and bottled water) is an absolute necessity. I drink so much water throughout a day that people who know me always tell me that at some point I will just float away. Since I work out every day, I very often drink about 3 liters of water every day (filtered and alkaline), in the summer it can be even more.

Vegetables

Vegetables form the most important part of your Macrobiotic Diet. 30% of your plate should include vegetables, either raw or cooked, found locally and seasonally. Green leafy vegetables are a must! An interesting fact is that the Macrobiotic Diet tells you not to include spinach, but it is something that I personally disagree with. I love spinach and spinach loves me. Besides, I also follow the Alkaline Diet, and as you may know, spinach is super alkalizing. It's up to you if you decide to "spinach it up!". Just my thoughts.

Soup

Soups are an essential component of this diet. They should be eaten daily to ensure maximum benefit from your macro meal. Soups that contain vegetables, grains, beans, and sea vegetables are ideal for a macro meal. Soups containing miso can also be eaten.

Fresh Fish (if you are not vegetarian/vegan)

A Macrobiotic Diet can also contain fish though this is entirely optional. If you are a vegetarian then you can skip this without it affecting your health in any manner. But for a non-vegetarian, white meat fish can be eaten 1-2 times in a week.

Fermented Foods

Tempeh and pickled vegetables are included in a Macrobiotic Diet.

<u>To be avoided:</u>

For a Macrobiotic Diet, there are some foods that you should steer clear of, or eat in moderation. These include:

- Any food containing refined sugar
- Artificial sweeteners
- Fruit juice, especially artificial and tropical fruits (unless you live in a hot, tropical climate)
- Caffeine (you won't need it when you start your Macrobiotic adventure)
- Refined oils
- Alcohol
- White rice and white flour
- A lot of spices
- Foods containing chemicals, insecticides, preservatives
- Milk, cream, butter, cheese, ghee, ice cream, and yogurt

An interesting fact: The above-mentioned items are considered to be acid forming in the Alkaline Diet.

A FEW WORDS ON FRUITS:

- What the Macrobiotic Diet says:

  Fruits should be avoided in a Macrobiotic Diet *though not altogether. You can eat them but not more than 3 times a week and tropical fruits like pineapple and banana should be altogether avoided.*

- What I do /my personal experience: I love fruits and I eat them, however I know what works for me and what not. Years ago, I would eat way too much fruit as I thought it was always good for me. The result was that I would very often feel bloated. This is how I react when I have too much fruit. I finally came to conclusion that what works well for me are seasonal fruits only, plus I tend to have more fruits in the summer. I seldom eat tropical fruits. I love a piece of fruit first thing in the morning, or in the afternoon. The Macrobiotic Diet does not recommend eating fruits as a dessert; it's better to have it as a quick snack. In my case, fruits satisfy my sweet tooth and I also grab a piece of fruit to have immediately when I go to or leave the gym. Try to see what works for you and your body. It's all that matters.

Many Macrobiotic and Alkaline Diet gurus will tell you to eliminate fruits and I am sure it may work for some people, but not for everyone. Personally, I think that fruits are healthy, natural, and refreshing.

On the Alkaline Diet, according to some "strict alkaline charts" most fruits (apart from limes, lemons, avocados, and tomatoes) are acid forming. What I learned and tested was that tropical fruits don't agree with me in large amounts (occasional tropical fruit desserts and smoothies are fine), but at the same time I am not able to eliminate or drastically reduce my intake of fruit. My body asks for it and I know that it works for my body. I restore my energy with fruit. I can't live without fruit.

My tip for you- see what works for you. I know people who thrive on a fruitarian style diet. It all comes down to testing and observing. Then, you should also take into account your geographical location. Just find your own balance, there is no need to reject fruit (again, this is my personal opinion).

And one more thing- before making any drastic changes to your diet, I suggest you consult your physician.

In the summer, I love fruit spa water. So, if you are concerned about intake of fruit (yes, many gurus will tell you how they contain sugar that is bad for you, but in my opinion, it's good, natural sugar that we also need every now and then, so if you are not suffering from any medical condition that prevents you from eating fruit, I don't see any problem), fruit infused water may be a solution for you (I have written a book called *Fruit Infused Water* if you want to check it out).

Finally, let's dive into the recipe section.

*As you will see, each recipe has "star-like hash tags", for example: *snack, *breakfast, *vegan....etc. so that you can make a quick selection depending on what you are looking for.*

Recipe Measurements

I love keeping ingredient measurements as simple as possible- this is why I stick to tablespoons, teaspoons and cups.

The cup measurement I use is the American cup measurement. I also use it for dry ingredients. If you are new to it, let me help you:

If you don't have American Cup measures, just use a metric or imperial liquid measuring jug and fill your jug with your ingredient to the corresponding level. Here's how to go about it:

1 American Cup= 250ml= 8 fl.oz

For example:

If a recipe calls for 1 cup of almonds, simply place your almonds into your measuring jug until it reaches the 250 ml/8oz mark.

I know that different countries use different measurements and I wanted to make things simple for you.

Your Unique Recipes

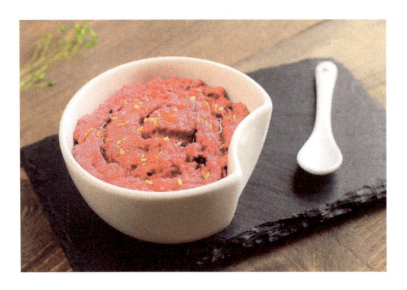

Beetroot Pudding

*vegan #gluten-free *vegetarian *breakfast *snack *energy

Serves: 3

Ingredients:

- 2 cups peeled and shredded beetroot

- 1 tablespoon coconut oil

- 2 tablespoons of almond butter

- 1 cup almond milk

- ¾ teaspoon cardamom powder

- ¼ teaspoon nutmeg powder

- 7-8 chopped almonds

- 7-8 chopped cashews

- ¼ cup raisins

Method:

1. Heat the coconut oil in a large sauce pan. Cook the shredded beetroot for about 12-15 minutes on low heat with the lid covered. Give it an occasional stir.

2. Add cardamom powder, almond milk and butter, nutmeg powder, raisins and cook for another 10-12 minutes on low heat. Remember to cover the saucepan with a lid. Stir occasionally.

3. Once the mixture cools down, refrigerate it for 60-90 minutes.

4. Heat another sauce pan and slightly roast the chopped almonds and cashews.

5. Garnish the beetroot pudding with toasted almonds and cashews on top.

6. Serve chilled.

Enjoy!

Pecan Granola

*breakfast *energy *vegan *vegetarian *sweet tooth *snack

Ingredients (for 12 granolas):

- 3 cups of regular rolled oats
- 1 /4 cup of pecans
- 1 teaspoon ground ginger
- 1 tablespoon Ceylon cinnamon
- 1/3 cup brown rice syrup
- 1/4 cup sesame or grape seed oil
- 2 pinches of sea salt
- 1/2 cup dried fruits like currants, dried apricots, raisins (optional)

Preparation:

1. Set oven to 300F.(150 Celsius)
2. Take a baking mold and smear it with a bit of oil.
3. In a bowl, mix oats, cinnamon, ginger and pecans, and in another bowl mix brown rice syrup, salt, and oil.
4. Pour the wet mix into the dry mix and blend well. Pour the mixture onto baking mold. .
5. Bake for about an hour.

6. Take it out of the oven. If you are using dried fruits, add it to the granola and stir. Otherwise, let it settle and then break into pieces.

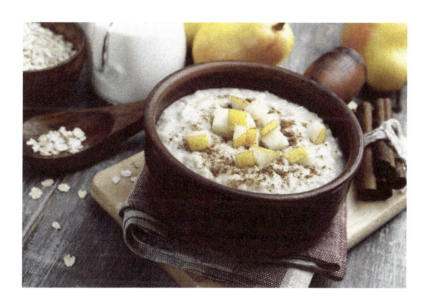

Creamy Whole Oats

*breakfast *energy *vegan *vegetarian *sweet tooth *snack

Ingredients (for 6 servings):

- 2 cups of oats
- 6 cups of water
- For toppings, choose from sunflower seed, butter, fruit jam, ground flax, raisins, cinnamon, maple syrup, flax oil.

Preparation:

1. Take a bowl and add water to it in the ratio of 3:1 with the amount of oats you are using. Let the oats soak overnight.

2. Take a pressure cooker and put the oats in it with some water and let it come to high pressure. Cook for about half an hour.

3. Spread it in a plate or in separate bowls to serve and add toppings as per choice.

Quick Oatmeal/Bran

*breakfast *energy *vegan *vegetarian *sweet tooth *snack

Ingredients (for one serving):

- 1/4 cup of oat bran
- 1/4 cup of rolled oats
- A cup of boiling hot water
- Coconut milk, cinnamon, cocoa nibs for toppings

Preparation:

1. Take up a coffee mug and add the oat bran and rolled oats to it.

2. Add the boiling water to it slowly, stirring it simultaneously.

3. Cover the mug using a lid to let the heat cook the oats.

4. Uncover the mug and add the toppings.

5. You may experiment by first putting hot cocoa in the empty cup as a base.

6. Enjoy!

Buckwheat Chia Oats

*breakfast *energy *vegan *vegetarian *sweet tooth *snack

Ingredients (for 1 serving):

- ¼ cup of buckwheat cereal
- 2 cups of water
- Salt as per taste
- 2 tablespoons of oat bran
- 2 tablespoons of Chia seeds
- Cinnamon, fresh blueberries (if in season), cashews, or maple syrup, etc. for toppings

Preparation:

1. Sprinkle a little salt to 1.5 to 2 cups of water. Bring the water to a quick boil.

2. Add buckwheat cereal to it and stir.

3. Cover it half with the lid, and allow it to simmer for about 5 minutes. Keep stirring it so that it is cooked evenly.

4. Add oat bran and Chia seeds to it and stir again.

5. Cook it for about 5 more minutes, bringing it to a very light boil. Add about half a cup of water to it at this point.

6. Take a bowl and pour the liquid into it. Allow it to cool. Cover it with your favorite topping. Enjoy!

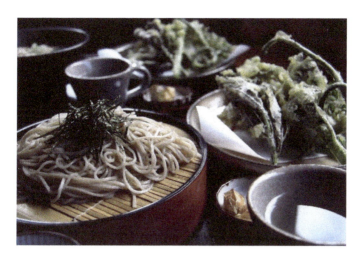

Sesame Vegetable Soba

*breakfast *lunch *brunch *vegan *natural protein

Ingredients (for 2 servings):

- 2 bundles of soba noodles
- 6 cups water
- Some pinches of sea salt
- 2 tablespoon of arrowroot powder or kuzu (for a slight thickening)
- Sesame oil
- 1 tablespoon of toasted sesame seeds
- 2 small carrots sliced in rounds
- Broccoli (finely chopped)
- 2 inches of Daikon, sliced in thin half moons
- Grated ginger to taste or 1 tablespoon ginger juice
- Firm pressed tofu (quantity according to 2 servings), cut finely and marinate in lemon juice, sesame oil along with shoyu for about an hour.
- Tamari

Preparation:

1. Add a pinch of salt to water and boil. Add noodles and cook for 5-6 minutes.

2. Scoop the noodles out and rinse in cold water. Remove the remaining water carefully. Keep the water in which you cooked your noodles.

3. Mix arrowroot powder or kuzu with very little water so that lumps are gone.

4. Add ginger juice and kuzu to the noodle water and stir. Put it to boil again and then let it simmer.

5. Sauté the vegetables in sesame oil with a lid until they are just soft. Add a little water if the vegetables are too dry. Add the vegetables to the broth from step 4.

6. Add tamari or shoyu to the broth and let it simmer for a minimum of 5 minutes.

7. Add oil/water (as convenient) to a pan and sauté tofu in it until it is evenly browned on each side.

8. Add the browned tofu to the vegetables and broth and simmer it for about 3 minutes.

9. Put the noodles into 2 bowls.

11. Add the vegetables and tofu into each bowl and pour the broth over the top in the two.

Yellow Split Pea Soup

*breakfast *lunch *brunch *vegan *gluten-free

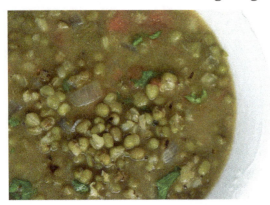

Ingredients (for 2 servings):

- 2 cups of yellow split peas (rinse and soak them for a while and drain)
- 3 cups of chopped greens, like kale
- 1 teaspoon of cumin and a small quantity of cayenne
- Flax seeds, parsley, sunflower seeds for toppings
- Salt, to taste
- 6 cups of water

Preparation:

1. Add the rinsed split peas to water and bring to boil. (You may scoop off the foam that forms)

2. Put it on low heat and allow it to simmer for about half an hour.

Alternately, you may simmer until the split peas appear to have broken down.

3. Add the chopped greens and cook until they are soft (for about 15 minutes).

4. Add spices and salt to taste and cook for around 10 more minutes.

5. Take some vegetables out and blend them before adding them back in the soup for thickness. Reheat.

6. Pour into a soup bowl and add the toppings.

French Lentil Stew

*lunch *dinner *vegan *natural protein *gluten-free

Ingredients (for 4 servings):

- 1.5 cups rinsed French lentils
- 1 cup diced carrots
- 1/2 cup sliced celery
- 1/2 finely diced ginger
- 1 cup diced parsnip
- 1.5 cups loosely packed parsley
- 1 tablespoon ground coriander
- 1 teaspoon dried thyme
- 4 cups boiling water
- 1 teaspoon sesame oil
- salt or tamari to taste
- lemon juice (optional)

Preparation:

1. Put the heat on medium and place the pressure cooker over it. Add oil.

2. Sauté the vegetables adding in this sequence: ginger, celery, carrots, and parsnips. Total sauté time should be around 3 minutes.

3. Add spices, sauté for 1 more minute while stirring.

4. Add boiling water.

5. Add lentils and stir. Lock the pressure cooker with lid and turn on high heat.

6. When the pressure is high, bring the heat to the lowest, and let it cook for 12 minutes.

7. Release the pressure and take off the lid.

8. Add salt and parsley and cook for 4 minutes while stirring.

9. Turn the heat off and serve with a lemon squeeze.

10. Enjoy!

Crust Less Pumpkin Pie

*healthy snack *vegan *lunch *brunch *breakfast *dinner

Ingredients:

- Organic pumpkin puree
- 1 heaping TBSP Kuzu Powder
- 1.5 cups rice milk or other dairy-free milk of your choice
- 2 Chia "eggs" (2 tablespoons white Chia seeds, whisked into and soaked in 7 tablespoons of water for 10 minutes)
- 3/4 cup maple or coconut palm sugar
- 1 teaspoon vanilla
- 1/2 cup oat
- 1/2 teaspoon nutmeg
- 1/2 teaspoon ground cloves
- 2 heaping teaspoon cinnamon
- A pinch of sea salt
- 2 teaspoon baking powder (aluminum free)
- Coconut or tofu whipped cream (for topping)

Preparation:

1. Set oven to 350F.(180 Celsius)

2. Mix every dry ingredient, except for the kuzu powder.

3. Blend Chia "eggs", dairy-free milk and vanilla. Add kuzu powder. Blend on high.

4. Add the pumpkin puree and again blend on high.

5. Add the dry ingredients and blend on high (1-2 minutes), until properly combined.

6. Oil a pie pan and pour the content of the blender.

7. Bake for about 60 minutes.

8. Let it cool before serving.

9. Serve with tofu or coconut whipped cream.

Brown Rice with Kimchi (Korean style)

*vegetarian * lunch *dinner *vegan

Ingredients (for one serving):

- Some cooked brown rice (1-2 cups)
- 2-3 heaping tablespoon Kimchi
- Soy sauce
- 1 tablespoon sesame seeds
- Cooking oil
- Mirin (rice cooking wine)
- Tofu, chopped and stir-fried in coconut oil

Preparation:

1. Put a pan on heat and add some cooking oil.

2. Put in brown rice and cook for around 3 minutes.

3. Add a splash of soy sauce and cook until it is absorbed.

4. Add some mirin and again cook until absorbed.

5. Add tofu on top and stir properly to mix.

6. Let it cook for a few minutes, then add Kimchi.

7. Add the sesame seeds and serve.

Delicious Rice Curry

*spicy *dinner *romantic *vegan

Ingredients (for 8 servings):

- 2 onions
- 2 red chili peppers diced
- 2 cubed red peppers
- Baby corns
- Green beans
- Garlic cloves-4
- broccoli
- 4 cubes of carrots
- 4-6 tablespoons of coconut cream
- 800 ml coconut milk (about 3 cups)
- Thai curry paste which is sugar free-2 - 3 tablespoons
- Herb salt
- Sesame oil
- Grated ginger
- Fresh lime juice,
- Coriander

Preparation:

1. Sauté the chili first. After the chili you can move on to sautéing the onions. Do all this in sesame oil. Add the pepper, carrots and finally a little bit of the garlic and stir. Put the Thai curry paste and mix.

2. Add the ginger, coconut cream and coconut milk. Then add the other vegetables, lime juice, and herb salt.

3. Stir occasionally and simmer it for 20 minutes, until all the vegetables are cooked. Add freshly chopped coriander.

4. For the yellow rice rinse the 2 cups of long grain rice, add 4 cups of water, salt, and turmeric. Then bring to a boil and simmer it for 20 minutes.

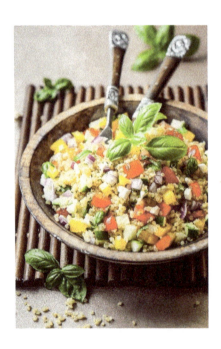

Delicious Rice from the Wilds

*vegan *lunch *dinner

Serves-1

Ingredients:

- Wild rice (about 1 cup)
- 3 cups water
- Sea salt (2 pinches to taste)
- Soy sauce
- Half onion. Cut in rings
- 1 small piece of alga wakame (about 2 square inches), soaked in water for about 15 mins
- 1 red pepper, minced
- 1 lime

Preparation:

1. Take a medium saucepan and put rice and water in it. Place the lid over the saucepan and then bring it to a boil.

2. Lower the flame to medium or lower and allow it to cook for three fourths of an hour.

3. Take away the lid and increase the flame. After which, it should cook for close to 5-6 minutes so that it is dry and no water is retained. Set aside.

4. In the meantime, sauté onion in some olive oil or coconut oil. When slightly brownish, add a few splashes of soy sauce. Keep sautéing and add the red pepper.

5. When the pepper is soft, add the rice and stir well so that it absorbs the aroma. Finally, cut alga wakame in small squares and add to the mix.

6. Serve with a few drops of fresh lime juice. Garnish with a slice of lime.

Stunning Black Eyed Beans

*vegan *lunch *dinner * natural protein

Ingredients (Serves 3):

- 2 cooked cups of black eyed beans
- 1 red pepper juliennes
- 1 yellow pepper juliennes
- Carrots juliennes
- Parsley
- Herb salt,
- Sesame oil

Preparation:

1. Get the sesame oil hot in a wok and fry the carrots and peppers.
2. Throw in the beans and add salt according to taste.
3. Add parsley and stir well.
4. Serve with some brown rice or basmati rice (excellent combination!).

Onions Complimenting Adzuki Beans

*lunch *dinner * vegan *natural protein

Ingredients (Serves 4):

- 2 cups of aduki beans, soaked in water for about 8 hours
- Alga Kombu cut into strips, at least 2
- 6 sliced onions
- Shoyu
- Brown rice (about 4 cups), soaked in water for about 8 hours
- Powdered sesame
- Parsley

Preparation:

1. Take the beans out of the water and clean them.
2. Place the rinsed beans in a pressure cooker with Kombu and 6-8 cups of water.
3. Bring up to pressure and cook for 45 minutes.
4. In the meantime, cook the brown rice (it should take max 20 minutes if the rice is properly soaked).
5. Heat up some sesame oil in a pot and sauté the onions. Add the cooked beans to the pot. Evaporate all the remaining water. Once you have a nice stew-like consistency, add the shoyu and rice syrup.

6. Add brown rice and stir well.

7. Serve this along with chopped parsley and sesame powder. Enjoy!

Tekka with Hot Brown Rice

*lunch *dinner *Asian *vegan *vegetarian

Ingredients (Serves 4):

- 1 cup minced onions
- 1 cup minced carrots
- 1 cup minced burdock
- 1 cup minced lotus root
- 4 tablespoons sesame oil or coconut oil
- 2 tablespoons Barley Miso diluted in water
- 2 spoons of grated ginger
- 1 spoonful of orange rind
- 2 cups of cooked brown rice

Preparation:

1. Heat oil in a pan.

2. Sauté the vegetables- onions, carrots, lotus root and burdock. Add water so that the vegetables are fully covered.

3. Cover the vegetables with a lid and simmer on a low flame until they are soft.

4. Add the diluted miso and cook for 3 minutes.

5. Add the orange rind and ginger and serve over hot brown rice. Enjoy!

Mushrooms with Spaghetti

*dinner *lunch *vegan *vegetarian *Italian

Ingredients (Serves 2):

- Spelt spaghetti
- Mushrooms
- A clove of garlic
- 1 diced onion
- Oat cream in a packet-1/2
- Herb salt
- Sesame oil

Preparation:

1. First cook spelt spaghetti as per instructions and put aside.
2. Heat some sesame oil in a pan to sauté the onions. Also add the crushed garlic and sauté.
3. Then add sliced mushrooms and herb salt.
4. Wait for the mushrooms to be soft after which you must add oat cream.
5. Add some spring onions & herb salt.
6. Add some freshly chopped parsley and serve with spaghetti. Enjoy!

Amazing Tempeh of Amasake

*vegan *vegetarian *lunch *dinner *dinner party *oriental

Ingredients (Serves 4):

- 2 blocks of Tempeh
- 4 tablespoons of amasake
- 6 medium onions (thinly sliced)
- 2 tablespoon of dried parsley
- 4 cloves of crushed garlic
- 4 tablespoons of water
- 4 tablespoons of shoyu

Preparation:

1. Slice up the Tempeh in any shape you want.
2. Place Tempeh, add water and shoyu in a baking tray. Evenly coat the Tempeh. Allow this mixture to rest for 15 minutes.
3. Slice the onions and crush the garlic. Take a frying pan, pour a little water and bring it to a boil.
4. Then add the garlic along with chopped onions. Let the mixture cook for about 8-10 minutes on low-medium heat. Then add in the amasake, parsley and Tempeh (with the liquid). Cover this and simmer it for 20 minutes.

5. Shoyu or seasoning can be added to the dish along with fresh parsley and sesame seeds or powder.

6. Enjoy!

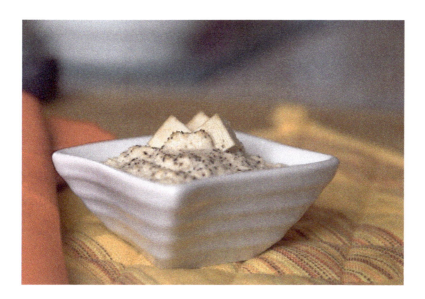

Onion Tempeh with Apricot

*vegan *vegetarian *lunch *dinner *snack

Ingredients (Serves 4):

- 2 blocks of Tempeh cut into cubes

- A few Apricots (soaked for 15 minutes)

- 4 onions (finely diced)

- 2-4 crushed garlic cloves (preferable)

- Shoyu (6-8 tablespoons)

- Concentrate of organic juice (apple juice preferably; about 4 tablespoons)

- 2 finely sliced leek

- Parsley

- Sesame oil/olive oil/ coconut oil

- Sunflower oil (will be used to deep fry)

Preparation:

1. To deep fry, heat the sunflower oil and fry the Tempeh.
2. Place the deep fried Tempeh in a bowl. Then, marinate the Tempeh with 6 tablespoons of shoyu and 4 tablespoons of the concentrate of apple juice. Stir occasionally.

3. Take a pan and pour sesame oil. Heat it. Then, take the sliced onions and add them to the oil. Allow the onions to cook until they are soft. This should take about 15 minutes.

4. Take out the apricots from the water and chop them. Apricots, garlic and the leek are to be added now to this mixture.

5. Add some water so as to cover the apricots and the onions. Cook for about 10 more minutes till the time the water evaporates.

6. Then put in the Tempeh, concentrate of apple juice and shoyu. If you feel the need, then you can add more shoyu. Cook until almost all of the liquid evaporates.

7. Put in chopped parsley and serve.

8. Enjoy!

Macrobiotic Seitan Paella

*vegan *lunch *dinner

Ingredients:

- 4 cups of short grain brown rice -washed & soaked for 2 hrs.
- 24 cups vegetable stock w/ Kombu
- 2 tsp. saffron
- ½ cups of olive oil
- 1 cup Seitan -cut into ¼ inch cubes
- Salt and pepper
- 2 cups of onion -medium dice
- 1/2 cup of carrot diced
- 1/2 cup of celery diced
- 4 tbs. Garlic –minced,
- 1/2 cup of summer squash sliced
- 2 cups of mushroom sliced
- 1/2 cups of burdock diced
- Parsley
- 4 lemons –quartered

Preparation:

1. Prepare the vegetable stock by using vegetable scraps & Kombu.

2. Heat the olive oil and sauté onions & garlic, stirring for 10 min.

3. Add the rice & saffron and cook for 10 more minutes while stirring constantly.

4. Add vegetable stock slowly while stirring, adding more stock as the rice absorbs. Continue adding the vegetable stock for 30 minutes on reduced heat.

5. Add carrot, celery, Seitan & burdock. Add more stock and keep on stirring for approximately 20 minutes.

6. Add mushrooms & squash while adding more stock and stirring.

7. Season it with pepper and salt and cook 10 more minutes.

8. Serve with chopped parsley and lemon wedges.

Delicious Corn on the Cob

*snack *vegan *quick prep

Ingredients (serves 1):

- 1 corn with cob (organic)
- Umeboshi paste/puree (a macrobiotic seasoning)
- Sesame powder

Preparation:

1. Boil the corn with cob in salty water. Do not roast.

2. Spread the Umeboshi paste and serve with sesame powder.

Macrobiotic Popcorns

*snack *vegan

Ingredients (serves 1):

- Handful of popping-corns
- 2 teaspoon. sesame oil
- 1 tablespoon peanut butter
- 1 tablespoon apple juice concentrates
- 2 tablespoon malt syrup or agave
- Pinch of Himalaya salt.

Preparation:

1. Take a pan and add the sesame oil with the corn kernels into it.

2. Place the lid on and increase the heat.

3. After a while the oil will heat and the corns will begin to pop up.

4. Check for slower popping (around 1 pop in 2 seconds). This way you'll know when it's ready.

5. Remove from heat and transfer the corns into a small bowl. Allow it to cool.

6. Now put the popcorn back into the cooking pot. Add all the other ingredients.

7. Ensure that the popcorn is still a bit moist (neither too sticky nor too dry). If it is too dry, fix it by adding some malt syrup.

8. Now give it a good mix and allow it to cool for some

time.

9. Serve and enjoy.

Green Sauerkraut Nori Starters

*vegan *lunch *dinner

Ingredients (serves 2):

- A medium sized carrot
- A lemon
- A bunch of radish
- Two sheets of nori
- Half a cup sauerkraut
- Spring greens or cabbage ,enough to fill the rolls
- Sea salt/Himalaya salt
- a fine bamboo mat

Preparation:

1. Wash the radish. Retain the green stalk, say half an inch.

2. Take a small pan and boil salted water in it. Now place the radish in this water to blanch it, once done remove the excess water.

3. Wash the carrot, grate it or cut it in extremely fine pieces and mix it with lemon juice.

4. Cut the greens into fine pieces.

5. Bring water to a quick boil, sprinkle a bit of salt and cook the vegetables until they are bright green.

6. Remove from heat and drain the water and strain hard, so that no water is left in it.

7. Take the sauerkraut and squeeze out excess juice,

place it on the cutting board and cut it very finely.

8. Wave the sheet of Nori over a low flame as instructed on its package. If you have a hot plate, gently hold the Nori sheet on it until the color changes.

9. Dry the prep board; place the mat in the center with the Nori. Place the non-shiny layer upwards.

10. Create a layer of all the greens, and then quarter way down, put down a thin line of sauerkraut. Roll up carefully and seal the edges.

11. Garnish and serve.

Creamy Macrobiotic Asparagus Soup

*vegan *vegetarian *warming *comforting

Ingredients (serves 1-2):

- 2 tablespoons of olive oil
- 4 carrots, sliced
- Chopped medium onion
- 1 leek with both parts (green and/or white) nicely diced
- 1 Japanese yam (chopped)
- Vegetable stock
- Sea salt
- 1 bunch of asparagus
- 1 tablespoon of dill (chopped)

Preparation:

1. Take a large sauce pan and pour olive oil into it and heat on medium.

2. Take the onions along with the leek and add to the pan. Sauté them for close to 5 minutes

3. Add the carrots and Japanese yam and continue sautéing for another 2 minutes.

4. Then add stock with 2 cups water and sprinkle about two tiny pinches of salt.

5. Bring the mixture to a boil. Then cover the pan and allow it to simmer till the time the vegetables are soft and tender. This should take a maximum of 20 minutes.

6. While the soup cooks, you should have the time to

start with the asparagus by taking out the lower halves of the stalks. Chop the tips and keep them aside. Cut the remaining stalks in lengths of about half an inch.

7. Take the soup pan off heat and allow it to cool down. Slowly add the chopped stems of the asparagus. Cover and leave until it cools down.

8. Put the soup into the blender in small batches. Allow it to blend till the time the mixture is smooth.

9. Now add the tips to the soup along with the dill and gently reheat.

Rice, Nut and Seed Roll

*vegan *dinner party *romantic

Ingredients (serves 4):

- Sesame oil
- 2 tablespoons ginger(grated)
- ½ cup of walnuts (soaked and chopped)
- 4 tablespoons of sunflower seeds (toasted)
- 4 tablespoons of pumpkin seeds (toasted)
- 2 tablespoon of sesame seeds
- 4 cups brown rice-cooked (short grain)
- Tamari (2 teaspoons or according to taste)
- 4 sheets of sushi seaweed (also called sushi Nori)

Preparation:

1. Take a small skillet and heat sesame oil in it. Then add ginger and sauté for about a minute.
2. Take the walnuts and all the seeds (sunflower, pumpkin, sesame) and add to the skillet. Along with this, add the rice.
3. Keep stirring thoroughly. After a while, add tamari.
4. Remove the skillet from heat and allow it to cool.
5. After the rice cools down, take one sheet of nori and spread half of the mixture on it.
6. Make sure that you spread the rice till the edges and be sure to leave a margin of about an inch on one side.

7. Now, keeping the cigar shape in mind, gently roll the nori and rice. Seal it by lightly applying a drop or two of water along the outside edge.

8. Repeat the same with the remaining rice mixture.

9. Serve hot. Enjoy!

Brown Rice & Hazelnut Balls

*dessert *sweet *vegan *energy

Ingredients (serves 2):

• Brown rice (Cooked; half cup)

• 1 teaspoon of hazelnut butter

• 1 tablespoon of rice syrup

• 1 tablespoon of toasted sesame seeds.

Preparation:

1. Blend all the ingredients.

2. Form into balls.

3. In case the mixture is still too wet, add rice but do not blend.

4. Take some nuts or seeds and/or powder (Coconut or carob) and roll the bolls in them for variety.

Apricot Mousse

*sweet *dessert *vegan *protein

Ingredients (serves 4):

- Apricots (dried; 2 cups)
- 1 cup of tofu, chopped
- 1 cup of water
- Rice milk (1 cup)
- Agar- agar seaweed
- A pinch of salt
- Orange juice (1 cup)
- Sesame/nut butter (1 tablespoon)
- Decoration: Almonds(roasted) & apricots (chopped)

Preparation:

1. Take a pan and put in some apricots and tofu. Add liquid ingredients and sprinkle a bit of salt. Boil the mixture.

2. The Agar-agar needs to be added now. Blend the mixture and put the pan on simmer for 20 minutes. Keep stirring.

3. Once done, blend the mixture. Make sure it is smooth in texture and add butter and mix.

4. Once the mixture cools down, put it in the refrigerator for a little over a half an hour so that it sets.

5. Then blend it again to attain a mousse like texture.

6. Serve with some cinnamon powder.

Adzuki Bean Truffles

*dessert *vegan *snack

Ingredients (serves 4):

- 1 cup of cooked adzuki beans
- 1 tbsp. of hazelnut butter
- 2 tbsp. of rice syrup
- Ground almonds
- A pinch of salt.

Preparation:

1. Mix the adzuki beans, rice syrup, vanilla, salt, hazelnut butter and enough ground almonds to knead dough that sticks and binds together.

2. Roll into small truffle sized balls.

3. Add a coating the way you please, treat yourself with these truffles with seasoning of grated coconut, coarsely chopped nuts and seeds, coco powder, sesame seeds or orange zest.

Blueberry Delight

*dessert *vegan

Ingredients (serves 4):

- Rice milk (3 cups)
- Agar flakes ½ cup
- Cinnamon
- Rice Syrup
- A pinch of salt
- Blueberries

Preparation:

1. Take a pan and pour rice milk into it.

2. Add agar flakes and sprinkle a pinch of salt and boil.

3. Keep the fire on and simmer the mixture like the time all the agar has dissolved.

4. For taste, you could add a bit of cinnamon and rice syrup.

5. Cool the mixture and serve it in glasses.

6. It could take close to an hour to set.

7. For the topping, take a pan and put some blueberries into it. Heat the berries until the time they are soft.

8. Add a pinch of salt and keep mixing till the mixture thickens. You could also add rice syrup for taste.

Mini Cranberry Tarts

*dessert *snack *vegetarian *yummy *sweet *vegan

Ingredients (serves 4):

FILLING:

- 2 cups of cranberries (fresh)
- 2 cups of apple/orange juice
- 1 tablespoon raisins
- 1 tablespoon orange/lemon zest.
- 1 tablespoon vanilla extract
- Half teaspoon cinnamon
- Half teaspoon ground cardamom
- Half teaspoon ground cloves
- Half tablespoon ginger (finely grated)
- Salt-to taste

PASTRY:

- 1 cup pastry flour (whole wheat)
- Two third cup flour (chickpea)
- Half cup olive oil
- Quarter cup syrup of brown rice
- Sea salt- to taste

Preparation:

To make the filling:

1. Take all the ingredients and add them to a pan and allow it to cook on low heat till the time the mixture is thick and a bit sticky.

2. In case the mixture is still too watery; you can add some kuzu to thicken.

3. In case if the mixture is too sour, then add barley malt to sweeten. You can also use brown rice syrup.

For the pastry:

1. Mix olive oil and rice syrup thoroughly.

2. Add the flours along with the salt in a small bowl and slowly pour the liquid into it till the time you get soft dough.

3. Kneading it a few times will help to bring it together.

4. Press it into tart tins of your choosing after you have oiled them.

5. Preheat the oven. Keep the temperature about 180 degrees Celsius or 350 Fahrenheit.

6. Bake the mixture for close to 20 minutes or until the time they are a good golden color.

7. Take it out and allow them to cool. After this, take the cranberry mixture and spread it in the tart case. Bake them for 5 minutes more.

8. They can be served with almond custard or oat cream.

Verdina Beans with Tofu

*lunch *dinner *vegan*vegan protein*algae

Ingredients (serves 2):

- 250g (1 cup) verdina bean (or any other bean if you can't find verdina, black beans are also great for this recipe)
- 2 square inches of kombu seaweed, cut
- 1 large onion, sliced
- 1 clove garlic, minced
- 1 maitake mushroom cut into flowers
- 1 "block" of smoked tofu, diced
- 3 cups of water
- 1 cup of vegetarian broth
- Extra virgin olive oil
- sea salt

Preparation:

1. Soak the beans for 8 hours.

2. Cook on low heat (mix water and vegetarian broth) with kombu seaweed for about 1 h. Add a few pinches of sea salt.

3. Sautee onion and garlic in some olive oil until soft and brownish. Set aside.

4. Now sauté tofu and maitake.

5. Add to the bean and kombu soup when almost ready. Turn off the heat.

6. Enjoy!

Variations:

- you can also add some quinoa or millet

Vegan "Meat" Balls

*vegan *dinner *lunch *spicy (if you want) *gluten-free

Ingredients (serves 2):
For the meatballs:

- 1 cup lentils (green or red)
- 1 piece of kombu seaweed (about 2-3 inches)
- 1 tablespoon of tahini
- 1 clove of garlic
- a few drops of lemon juice
- herbs and spices of your choice(I like to use curry with a bit of chili powder and a few pinches of rosemary herb)
- sea salt

For the stir fry:

- 1 onion
- 1 carrot
- Kelp seaweed noodles
- extra virgin olive oil
- sea salt

Preparation:

1. Wash the lentils and pressure cook with kombu seaweed and herbs for at least 1h.

2. Strain them and put the cooking water aside, you will need some of it.

3. Blend the lentils with a bit of cooking water, add the juice of ½ lemon and 1 teaspoon tahini, plus 1 clove garlic for more taste.

4. Slice the onion and a carrot. Make the slices super thin so that they match nicely with Kelp noodles.

5. Soak Kelp noodles in filtered water for about 5 mins.

6. Sauté the onions with a little olive oil and a pinch of salt. Add the carrot slices and continue to sauté. Add the seaweed with 2 tablespoons of "soaking water" (it's full of nutrients) and continue sautéing (use low heat) for about 10 mins.

7. Meanwhile, form lentil balls.

8. When the stir-fry is ready, turn the heat off. Place the veggies on a plate and add the vegan "meatballs" on top. Serve with a slice of lime or lemon.

Broccoli Rice

*lunch *dinner *vegan

Ingredients (serves 1-2):

- 1 cup red rice (boiled in two cups of water with a piece of kombu seaweed and cooled down)
- 1 avocado, peeled and cut into cubes
- 1 small piece of pumpkin cut into cubes
- The green part of 2 leeks, finely chopped
- broccoli cut into florets (about 1 cup)
- black olives, pitted (1 cup)
- rice milk or almond milk (1/4 cup)
- olive oil
- sea salt

Preparation:

1. Steam pumpkin, broccoli and leek for a few minutes, until soft.

2. In the meantime, make your mayonnaise: mix ¼ cup of vegan milk of your choice (e.g. almond) a few teaspoons of almond powder, a few pinches of salt and black pepper and a few drizzles of olive oil.

3. Mix the rice with the vegetables (except broccoli) and vegan mayonnaise and place in a fridge to cool down

4. Serve chilled, garnish with black olives, cut in halves and broccoli florets.

Refreshing Summer Leek Soup

*summer *cream *vegan *lunch *dinner

Ingredients (serves 4):

- 10 leeks stems (the green part)
- 1 onion, peeled and sliced
- 1 cup of oatmeal cream (can be also oat milk with some crashed cash nuts for more density) or coconut milk
- Extra virgin olive oil
- white miso (1 tablespoon)
- fresh dill
- 2 cups of water

Preparation:

1. Wash and slice the leek stems.

2. Sauté in a tablespoon of olive oil in a large pot. Add the onion.

3. Cover with 2 cups of water and boil for about 15 minutes. Add a few pinches of salt.

4. Add fresh dill, 1 cup of vegan cream of your choice, one tablespoon white miso and continue cooking for 2-3mn more, stirring.

5. Turn off the heat and blend the cream.

6. Cool down in a fridge and serve with a sprig of dill. Taste to see if you need any more salt or spices.

7. Enjoy!

Optional: I like to add some pistachios and raw carrot slices for more variety. This dish is also excellent with tofu and beans.

Macrobiotic Smoothie

*breakfast *snack *energy *vegan *vegetarian *alkaline
*gluten-free

Ingredients (serves 1):

- Half cup of cooked quinoa, cooled
- Alga wakame (about 3-4 cm 2), soaked in water for about 10 minutes
- 1 cup of almond milk
- Juice of 1 lemon
- 2 carrots, peeled and sliced
- A few raisins (to garnish)
- Half cup of kale

Preparation:

1. Mix all the ingredients in a blender.

2. Garnish with a few raisins. You can also blend them in if you want your smoothie to be sweet.

Kukicha Tea Energy!

*snack *breakfast * energy *vegan *vegetarian *gluten-free

Ingredients (serves 2):

- Half cup of raw almonds
- 1 cup of cooked amaranth
- 1 cup of almond milk
- 1 cup of kukicha tea, cooled
- 1 apple, peeled, pitted and sliced finely
- 1 carrot, peeled and sliced (make it really thin)
- A few drops of fresh lemon juice

Preparation:

1. Mix all the ingredients in a cereal/ muesli bowl.

2. Add a few drops of lemon juice.

3. Garnish with a slice of lemon.

4. Enjoy, this recipe is energy and life!

Green Adzuki Salad

*vegan *vegetarian *dinner *lunch *natural protein

Ingredients (serves 2-3):

- 3 cups of cooked and cooled integral rice (you can also use basmati rice)
- 1 cup of adzuki beans, cooked and cooled
- 1 cup of minced radish and chive
- A few drops of lemon juice and soy sauce
- Himalaya salt

For the salsa:

- 1 clove of garlic, peeled
- 1 big avocado, peeled, pitted and sliced
- 2 tablespoons of olive oil, coconut oil or grape seed oil
- Half cucumber, peeled
- 1 carrot, peeled (unless organic)
- Juice of 1 lemon

Preparation:

1. In a blender, mix all the ingredients from "for the salsa" part. Set aside.

2. In a separate bowl, mix rice, adzuki, radish, and chive.

3. Add salsa, mix well and season with Himalaya salt, soy sauce and lemon juice according to your personal taste.

4. So easy, quick and nutritious! Enjoy!

Simple and Quick Macrobiotic Basmati Rice

*vegan *vegetarian *dinner *lunch

Ingredients (serves 2-3):

- 3 cups of basmati rice, cooked
- 1 cup of cooked chickpeas, cooled
- 2 big green bell peppers, sliced finely
- Half onion, minced
- Coconut oil
- ¼ cup of sesame powder
- A few slices of alga kombu or wakame
- Lemon
- ¼ cup of vegetarian broth
- Soy sauce and Himalaya salt to taste

Preparation:

1. Soak algae in filtered water for about 15 mins.

2. In the meantime, steam the bell peppers until soft. Set aside on a separate plate and sprinkle over a few drops of lemon.

3. Sautee onion in coconut oil. When brownish, add sesame powder. Lower to low heat.

4. Add vegetarian broth, stir well, add basmati rice, alga and bell peppers. Mix well and turn off the heat.

5. Add a few drops of soy sauce and Himalaya salt to taste. Enjoy!

Energy Restoring Carrot Juice

*breakfast * quick energy *vegan *vegetarian *gluten-free

Ingredients (serves 1):

- 4 carrots, peeled and sliced
- 1 apple, peeled and sliced
- Half cup of quinoa, cooked
- Half cup of rice milk
- Half cup of water
- ¼ cup of agar-agar seaweed (soaked)
- 2 tablespoons of powdered sesame (to garnish)
- A slice of lime

Preparation:

1. Blend all the ingredients, including agar-agar.

2. Serve immediately. Garnish with a slice of lime and sesame powder.

Green Macrobiotic Easy Smoothie

*alkaline *vegan * vegetarian *snack *energy *detox *
breakfast *gluten-free

Ingredients (serves 1-2):

- 1 cup of almond milk
- 1 cup of roibosh tea (cooled)
- 1 cup of cooked amaranth
- Half cup of chopped broccoli florets (previously steamed until soft)
- Half cup of kale leaves
- ¼ cup raisins
- 2 teaspoons of chlorella powder
- Optional- stevia to sweeten (I usually do without it, raisins already make it sweet, but see what works for you)

Preparation:

1. Blend all the ingredients.
2. Shake and stir well before serving.
3. Garnish with a slice of lime.

Alkaline Macrobiotic Tofu Mix

*vegan *alkaline *protein *high energy levels *gluten-free

Ingredients (serves 2):

- 2 cups of broccoli florets, previously steamed until soft
- 2 garlic cloves, minced
- Half onion, minced
- 1 block of tofu
- 1 cup of radish
- 1 cup of kale leaves, finely chopped
- Half cup of almonds
- Once slice of alga wakame or kombu (about 2 square inches)
- Olive Oil
- Juice of 1 lemon
- 2 tablespoons of sesame powder
- ½ cup of cooked amaranth
- Soy sauce (go for gluten free)

Preparation:

1. Let alga kombu (or wakame) soak in water for about 15 minutes.
2. In the meantime, cut tofu into small slices and sauté in some olive oil with minced onion. Add a bit soy sauce so that tofu absorbs the flavor.
3. When slightly brownish, turn off the heat and set aside.
4. In a bowl, place steamed broccoli florets, kale, almonds, and radish. Add tofu.
5. In a separate glass or a mini bowl, mix 2 tablespoons of olive oil, some lemon juice (1 lemon), minced garlic, powdered sesame, amaranth, and a splash of soy sauce for more taste. Stir well.
6. Spread the salsa on the salad. Serve with a slice of lime or lemon on side.

Macrobiotic Green Alkaline Springtime Salad

During the springtime, the macrobiotic diet recommends to increase the consumption of green veggies as it helps to cleanse the liver and the gallbladder.

*vegan *vegetarian *energy *health

Ingredients (serves 2):

- 1 cup of radish, sliced
- 4 carrots, sliced
- 2 cucumbers, sliced
- 1 avocado, sliced
- About 2 square inches of alga wakame and kombu
- 2 cups of brown rice (cooked)
- Juice of 1 lemon
- Half onion, minced
- ¼ cup of chopped chive
- 2 tomatoes, sliced
- Olive oil

Preparation:

1. Let the algae soak in water for about 15 mins. You may want to chop the algae into small pieces before soaking them.
2. Mix all the ingredients, including the algae in a bowl.
3. Sprinkle over some olive oil and lemon juice.
4. Serve immediately.

Macrobiotic Sweet Apple Carrot Dip

*dessert *snack *vegan *gluten-free

Ingredients (serves 2):

- 5 big carrots, sliced
- 4 apples, peeled, cored and sliced
- ½ cup of agar-agar
- 2 tablespoons of cinnamon
- sesame powder
- coconut oil
- 1 cup of rice milk (gluten-free)
- 3 cups of water

Preparation:

1. Put water to boil. Add carrots, cinnamon, apples and agar-agar.
2. Turn off the heat when boiling. Add rice milk and stir well. Cover and let it cool down.
3. Finally, mix all the ingredients in a blender. Add sesame powder and coconut oil/milk for more consistency and taste.
4. Serve this dip with organic rice cakes or sesame bars. So yummy!

Chickpeas Easy Bread (gluten-free)

If you can't live without bread- make your own!

*vegan *vegetarian *snack * natural protein *gluten-free

Ingredients (makes 1 small bread):

- 1 cup of water
- 1 cup of chickpeas flour
- Herbs to taste: rosemary, thyme, and if you like it spicy- a bit of chili powder
- Himalaya salt

Preparation:

1. Preheat the oven to 180 Celsius degrees (350 Fahrenheit).

2. In the meantime, blend all the ingredients in a blender.

3. Spread the mixture onto a baking tray (smear with a bit of coconut oil or olive oil).

4. Bake for about 30- 40 minutes.

5. Serve with veggie dips of your choice.

Amazing Apple Salad

*vegan *snack *light lunch *quick prep

Ingredients (serves 1):

- 1 big apple
- 1 red chicory
- For the salsa: 1 tablespoon of lemon or lime juice + 1 tablespoon of olive oil + 1 tablespoon of organic apple juice
- Optional (I love it though): umeboshi vinegar to spice up the salsa
- A pinch of salt
- ¼ onion, cut into rings
- 1/ 4 cup of raisins

Preparation:

1. Mix all the ingredients in a bowl.
2. Add Salsa and umeboshi vinegar.
3. Garnish with a few raisins.

Really Easy and Quick Quinoa Salad

*vegan *quick prep *lunch *dinner

Ingredients (serves 2):

- 2 cups of quinoa, cooked
- 1 cup of radish
- 1 cup of snow peas, cooked
- Pinch of Himalaya salt
- Olive oil and umeboshi vinegar
- Slice of lime/lemon
- 1 tablespoon of sesame seeds powder

Preparation:

1. Mix all the ingredients in a bowl.
2. Add a splash of olive oil and umeboshi vinegar, according to your taste.
3. Garnish with a slice of lime or lemon and add sesame seeds powder.

Easy and Nutritious Bimi Meal

*quick prep *lunch *dinner *nutritious *gluten-free

Ingredients (serves 1-2):

- 250gr. (1 cup) of bimi (it is an exotic veggie similar to broccoli, if you can't find it, just use broccoli instead), chopped
- 1 onion, chopped
- 1 bulb of fennel, chopped
- Coconut oil
- Soy sauce (make sure it's gluten-free)
- 1 garlic clove, peeled and minced

Preparation:

1. In a pan, sauté the onion and garlic in a bit of coconut oil.
2. When slightly brownish add the rest of the ingredients together with a splash of soy sauce and a bit of water.
3. Lower the heat and keep simmering for about 15 minutes.
4. Optional: add a few raisins.
5. Serve slightly warm, or chilled, for example on brown rice or quinoa.

Vegan Burgers with Macrobiotic Dip

*vegan *burger *protein *lunch *brunch

Ingredients (serves 2):

- 2 cups cooked chickpeas
- 1 onion, minced
- 1 cup cooked corn or peas
- 1/2 cup chickpea flour
- a handful of sesame seeds
- For the dip: 2 onions and 6 carrots
- Olive oil and coconut oil

Preparation:

1. Blend chickpeas with onions and corn.
2. Form mini burgers and "coat them" with some sesame seeds and chickpea flour.
3. Fry them in some olive oil.
4. Serve the burgers with Macrobiotic dip: simply cook or steam carrots and onions and blend them with a bit of coconut oil and salt.

Millet Puree with Vegan Sausages

*gluten-free *vegan *protein

Ingredients (serves 2)

- a cup of millet, cooked
- 2 tablespoons of white miso
- 2 onions, minced
- 2 cups of mushrooms, diced
- 4 tofu sausages
- 1 teaspoon of kudzu
- ½ cup of snow peas

Preparation:

1. Mix millet with white miso and a bit of coconut or olive oil and blend.
2. Sautee the mushrooms with minced onions and when soft, put on top of millet pure.
3. Stir-fry the tofu sausages and serve with this dish. I like to garnish it with a bit of kale leaves and radishes.

Carrot Wakame Detox Soup

*vegan *vegetarian *detox *energy *gluten-free

Serves-4
Ingredients:

- 5 carrots, sliced
- 1 cup of coconut milk or almond milk
- 1 onion, peeled and chopped
- A few inches of wakame
- 1 cup of cooked amaranth
- Himalaya Salt to taste

Instructions:

1. Put water to boil and add carrots and onion.

2. Turn off the heat when the water starts boiling. Cover and let it cool down.

3. In the meantime, soak alga wakame in water for about 15 mins.

4. Finally, blend all the ingredients (including vegan milk) in a blender and add cooked amaranth (an excellent source of iron).

5. Serve chilled or re-heat. Season with Himalaya Salt

Variations:

Instead of carrots, you can also use peppers, zucchini, eggplant and cauliflower. Experiment with different spices and grains (for example millet, brown rice) as well as legumes that you can also add to your macrobiotic soup (I love adzuki beans especially in the winter).

Quinoa and Chickpea Curry

*vegan *protein *gluten-free *nutritious *oriental

This one is really recommended if you want to show your friends that a vegan-alkaline diet is actually exciting and fun!

Serves: 2

Ingredients:

- 1 cup quinoa

- 1 cup chickpeas (soaked overnight)

- 1 minced garlic clove

- 1 teaspoon minced ginger

- 5-6 chopped spinach leaves

- 1 tablespoon lemon juice

- ½ cup diced sweet potato cubes

- 2 chopped tomatoes

- 1 medium onion, chopped

- 2 cups vegetable broth

- 1 teaspoon garam masala

- 1 bay leaf

- 1 teaspoon salt

- 2 tablespoon coconut oil

- Some cilantro for garnishing

Method:

1. Heat some oil in a sauce pan. Sauté the garlic and onion for about 3-4 minutes.

2. Throw in the bay leaves, spinach, chopped sweet potato, quinoa and cook for 5-6 minutes

3. Add the soaked chickpea, followed by some salt, garam masala and vegetable broth. Cook this curry for about 15-16 minutes on medium flame. Remember to cover the saucepan with a lid.

4. Sprinkle some lemon juice on top.

5. Garnish with some cilantro. So yummy and healthy!

Vanilla Flavored Quinoa Porridge

*vegan *protein *gluten-free *nutritious *oriental

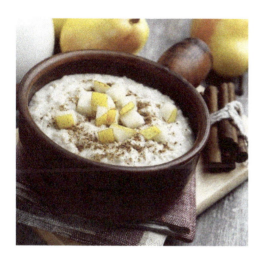

Serves: 3

Ingredients

- 1 cup quinoa

- 2 cups almond milk or coconut milk (don't count calories)

- 1 teaspoon vanilla essence or stevia (optional)

- ¼ cup chopped almonds

- ¼ teaspoon ground nutmeg

- ½ teaspoon cardamom powder

- 1 teaspoon freshly shredded ginger

- ¼ teaspoon salt

Method

1. Place some almond milk in a large vessel, add nutmeg powder, cardamom powder and bring it to a boil.

2. Add the quinoa; let it cook for about 12-15 minutes with the lid covered. Ensure that the quinoa is fully cooked.

3. Now throw in the shredded ginger, salt, vanilla essence, and let it simmer for about 7-8 minutes.

4. Once it cools down slightly, refrigerate this porridge for at least an hour before serving.

5. Heat a saucepan and slightly toast the chopped almonds on low heat.

6. Drizzle some over the quinoa porridge.

7. Serve slightly chilled (or nicely warm in the winter).

8. Enjoy! (I also like to add in some maca powder and cocoa for extra boost)

Spicy Thai Rolls

*vegan *protein *gluten-free *nutritious *oriental

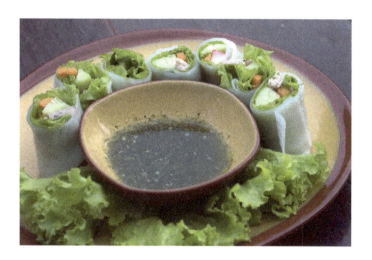

Serves: 4

Ingredients:

- 1 cup freshly shredded cabbage

- 1 cup freshly shredded carrot

- 1 sliced banana

- 8-10 chopped almonds

- 1 minced garlic clove

- 1 tablespoon sesame oil

- 1 tablespoons minced ginger

- 1 teaspoon chili flakes

119

- 2 teaspoons dried basil

- 10-12 Romanian lettuce leaves

- ¾ teaspoon Himalayan salt

- 1 tablespoon soy sauce or coconut oil infused with garlic and ginger (or both)

- 2 tablespoons soaked tamarind pulp

- 4 tablespoons pomegranate seeds

Method:

1. In a bowl, combine shredded carrot, cabbage, banana, ginger, garlic, pomegranate seeds, chili flakes, basil, tamarind pulp, soy sauce, sesame oil, salt and mix well. If you wish you can add some flax seeds to this mixture too.

2. Fill this mixture into each of the lettuce leaves gently and secure them with a toothpick.

3. Serve along with some mint sauce (*next recipe*)

4. Enjoy!

Tofu in Mint Sauce

*vegan *protein *gluten-free *nutritious *oriental

This recipe is extremely refreshing and alkaline! Make sure you choose good quality tofu though.

Serves: 4

Ingredients:

- 1 cup diced tofu
- ½ cup fresh mint leaves
- ½ cup coriander leaves
- 1 green chili
- 1 tablespoon lemon juice
- Pinch of Himalaya salt
- ½ teaspoon pepper
- 1 diced green bell pepper
- 1 diced red bell pepper
- 2 diced onions
- 1 cup cubed pineapple
- 1 tablespoon organic barbecue sauce
- ½ tablespoon oregano

- ½ teaspoon basil (dried)

- 2 tablespoons olive oil (or coconut oil)

- 3-4 skewers

Method:

1. Make a smooth paste of chopped mint, coriander, lemon juice, green chili and salt using a blender.

2. Coat the diced tofu in the mint sauce and set it aside for 60 minutes.

3. Heat some oil in a sauce pan. Sauté the onions and bell peppers for about 2-3 minutes. Switch off the flame.

4. Insert the diced onions, bell pepper, pineapple and marinated tofu onto a skewer.

5. Sprinkle some dried basil and oregano on it.

6. Heat some oil in a sauce pan and fry them for about 5-6 minutes on each side until they turn slightly brown.

7. Serve hot.

Asian Style Noodle Salad

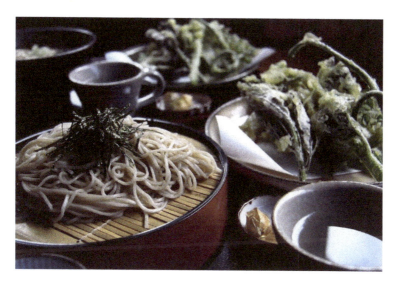

Serves: 3

Ingredients:

- 1 cup shitake or button mushrooms, chopped

- ½ cup chopped and blanched kale leaves

- ½ cup blanched broccoli florets

- 1 medium onion, sliced

- 2 tablespoons of olive oil

- ¾ teaspoon pepper

- ½ teaspoon salt

- ½ cup sprouts

- 1 teaspoon dark soy sauce (low sodium)

- 1 cup soba noodles

- About 2 cups water to boil the noodles

- Some chopped parsley for garnish

Method:

1. Take some water in a large sauce pan and bring it to a boil. Add half a teaspoon of olive oil so the noodles don't stick to each other.

2. Slide in the noodles and cook for about 3-4 minutes until they become slightly tender. Remember not to overcook the noodles. Drain the water. Set aside.

3. Take a salad bowl and mix the mushrooms along with kale leaves, broccoli florets, onion, noodles, pepper, salt, soy sauce and sprouts.

4. Drizzle some olive oil on top and toss.

5. Garnish with chopped parsley. Enjoy!

Macrobiotic Diet Recipes

Bonus Recipes- Super Healthy Smoothies (Alkaline, No Sugar, No Dairy, No Gluten)

Super high in nutrients and rich in natural protein. Perfect to help You enjoy more energy!

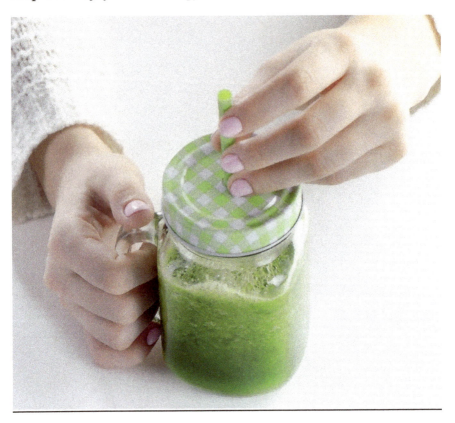

Creamy Protein Delight

This is one of my favorite super alkaline smoothies. It combines natural protein from chia seeds with good fats from avocado.

It's naturally creamy and beginner-friendly. Lemons (or limes) blend really well with avocados. This smoothie tastes a bit like Greek yoghurt but is fully plant-based and dairy free.

You can also serve this smoothie as a smoothie bowl, with some nuts and seeds (for example almonds and cashews).

Serves: 1-2

Ingredients

- 2 cups cold unsweetened coconut milk or almond milk
- 2 tablespoons chia seeds (or chia seed powder)
- 1 small lemon, peeled and sliced
- 1 small avocado, peeled and pitted
- a few lime slices to garnish
- a pinch of Himalayan salt

Instructions

1. Place all the ingredients in a blender.
2. Blend until smooth.

3. Pour into a smoothie glass, or serve in a small bowl with some nuts and seeds.

4. Enjoy!

Beautiful Skin Alkaline Protein Drink

People always ask me about natural beauty tips and the Alkaline Diet can surely help! My recommendation is to focus on what you eat (and drink) first.

In my twenties (especially my early twenties) I spent lots of money on magic solutions, creams and other shortcuts. However, it was only when I decided to take care of the inside and put my health first that the real transformation took place.

This is one of my favorite 100% alkaline smoothie recipes that combines the power of beta-carotene rich ingredients to help you have beautiful, healthy looking skin.

This smoothie is also very filling and nourishing! Oh, and needless to say it tastes creamy. I am not a big fan of those pitiful smoothies that taste like baby food and take lots of willpower to get through as well.

Serves: 1-2

Ingredients

- 1 cup coconut or almond milk
- Half cup coconut water
- 2 small carrots, peeled
- 1 big red bell pepper, cut into smaller pieces

- 2 tablespoons hemp seed protein powder
- 1 teaspoon cinnamon powder

Optional- stevia to sweeten if needed

Optional- fresh mint leaves and lime slices to serve

Instructions

1. Place all the ingredients in a blender.
2. Blend until smooth.
3. Pour into a glass and enjoy!

This smoothie is a fantastic way of adding more veggies to your diet, first thing in the morning.

Red bell peppers are one of my favorite alkaline superfoods. They are naturally sweet, inexpensive and very easy to find (even in your local grocery store).

No excuses- a healthy lifestyle doesn't have to be about overpriced supplements and complicated rituals.

Creating a healthy foundation is all about simplicity, and what you need is already within your reach.

Green Aroma Smoothie

Moringa is an alkaline superfood. It contains all the essential amino acids – the building blocks of protein- that are needed to grow, repair and maintain cells. At the same time, it's rich in alkaline forming minerals such as magnesium, iron and potassium.

Mint and cilantro give this smoothie a refreshing taste while adding a ton of micronutrients and antioxidants. They also aid in digestion. Perhaps you are not a big fan of spinach or kale smoothies, or maybe you are looking for new, original recipes. Well, the good news is that there are different options out there!

Serves: 1-2
Ingredients

- 1 cup almond milk
- A handful almonds, soaked in filtered water for at least a few hours
- 1 inch fresh ginger, peeled
- 1 teaspoon moringa powder
- A few avocado slices
- A handful fresh mint, washed
- A handful fresh cilantro leaves, washed

Instructions

1. Place all the ingredients into a blender

2. Process well until smooth.

3. Enjoy!

Lime Flavored Protein Smoothie

This smoothie is great as a quick energizing snack or even as a dessert. It uses stevia to create natural sweetness. It's also rich in healthy protein, good fats and vitamin C. Cinnamon and ginger add to its alkaline and anti-inflammatory properties.

Serves: 1-2

Ingredients

- 1 cup unsweetened coconut or almond milk
- 2 small limes, peeled and cut into smaller pieces
- 1 teaspoon cinnamon powder
- 1-inch ginger, peeled
- 1 tablespoon avocado oil
- 1 tablespoon chia seeds
- Optional: stevia to sweeten

Instructions

1. Place all the ingredients in a blender.
2. Process well until smooth.
3. If needed, sweeten with stevia.

Serve in a smoothie glass and sprinkle some cinnamon powder on top for extra sweetness.

Final Thoughts

I want to thank you once again for taking an interest in my work. It really means a lot to me, I hope you are getting ready to cook at least a couple of my delicious and healthy recipes. Trying to eat more macrobiotic, is one thing you would never regret. Try it for about a month and experience the wonders of this diet yourself.

Finally, remember that it's not about perfection, it's about progress, try to do the best you can and keep moving forward. Taking imperfect action and learning on the way is better than not doing anything. I wish you all the best on your wellness journey!

Marta

www.HolisticWellnessProject.com

PS. *One more thing, before you go, I need to ask you a favor. Could you please honestly rank this book on Amazon and post a short review? Your comments are very important to me. It's you I am writing for and I would love to hear from you. What was your favorite recipe/ wellness tip you got from this read?*

Thank You in advance!

Want to Stay in Touch?

The best way to stay in touch is via my Alkaline Wellness Email Newsletter you can join at no cost at: www.holisticwellnessproject.com/alkaline

As soon as you sign up you will receive free instant access to 3 VIP Bonus Guides to help you on your journey.

3 Free Bonus Guides

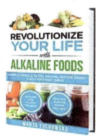 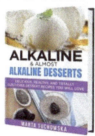 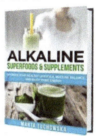

If you happen to have any problems with your download, email me at:
info@holisticwellnessproject.com

More Wellness Books by Marta

www.HolisticWellnessProject.com/books

www.amazon.com/author/mtuchowska

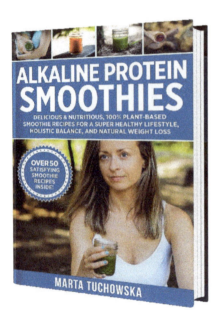

CPSIA information can be obtained
at www.ICGtesting.com
Printed in the USA
LVHW070816280420
654614LV00018BB/1015